Health Care R

**Health and Nursing Studies for
Diploma and Undergraduate Students**

Health Psychology
Authors: Glenys Pashley and I C Henry

Health Ethics
Authors: I C Henry and Glenys Pashley

Health Care Research
Authors: I C Henry and Glenys Pashley

**Health and Nursing Studies for
Diploma and Undergraduate Students**

Health Care Research

by

I C Henry and Glenys Pashley

Quay Publishing
11 Victoria Wharf
St George's Quay
Lancaster LA1 1GA

British Library Cataloguing in Publication Data
Henry, I.C. 1946–
        Health care research. (Health and nursing studies
        for diploma and undergraduate students, 3).
        1. Psychology
        I. Title II. Pashley, Glenys 1955 III Series
        150
ISBN 1-85642-003-5 1990

©   Henry I C and Pashley G

All rights reserved. No part of this publication may be reproduced, stored in a retrieval system, or transmitted in any form or by any means, electronic, mechanical, photocopying, recording or otherwise, without prior permission from the publishers.

Printed in Great Britain by Butler and Tanner Limited, Frome, Somerset.

Contents

Prelims		i–vi
1	What is health care research?	1
2	Types of research	11
3	The ethical issues of research	16
4	Preparation and design for completing research	23
5	The questionnaire	33
6	The interview	43
7	Action research	52
8	The case study	60
9	Triangulation	67
10	Critical evaluation of research articles	74
11	Further reading on research methods	79
Index		87

Chapter 1

What is health care research?

Health care research is concerned with the extension of knowledge regarding health-related issues, and this may involve the person in terms of his/her biology, and/or psychology and/or social features. In one sense, these features are interdependent and, therefore, render some forms of applied research difficult, especially when researchers are attempting to focus on one or two particular aspects. Researching the effects of stress on nurses working in an intensive care unit, for example, is complex and it is difficult to separate the influential factors; physiological symptoms of stress may or may not be exacerbated by how the individual nurse psychologically perceives and interprets his/her social working environment. Nevertheless, health care research seeks to increase our understanding and to provide some kind of explanation for whatever is the chosen topic of study. Central to this search for knowledge, understanding and explanation is the term 'generalisation'. Understanding something demands that we can relate one idea to another, compare instances, search for patterns, form expectations and make predictions. In other words, we feel we know something when we can generalise. Generalisation may well be a common aim for all research, but it is essential to acknowledge that different approaches place different levels of emphasis upon the necessity to generalise. The question arises, "How far can we generalise about the person, health and illness?" The term 'person' is not the same as a thing or an object; it is species neutral and more appropriate for the social sciences than the natural sciences.

Research is linked to the notion of science; a method of approaching and studying phenomena in an objective, systematic and controlled way, and one that has been very much dependent upon observation and quantitative or statistical analysis. There is a need, however, to balance this quantitative approach with a qualitative approach, and this encourages the potential for diverse and varied research topics in health care. Examples include, health professionals' attitudes towards the care of the critically ill, conceptions of mental illness as seen by psychiatric and/or general nurses, or investigations concerning the number of women who experience postnatal depression. It is important to note that the latter example is more quantitatively based and, therefore, more amenable to the scientific approach. Further, the researcher might be concerned with identifying, on a national and/or regional and/or district level, the number, age and whether the women aremore likely to be single parents or not. This is a fairly simplistic example of research that essentially deals in numbers, involves the collection of empirical data and some level of statistical analysis. This type of research fits with a scientific or positivistic approach and also links closely to the kind of research carried out by the natural sciences, taken to include disciplines like chemistry, physics and biology. In chemistry, certain compounds of liquids can be observed, changes can be measured and laboratory experiments easily repeated. Similarly, in biology, a human organ can be dissected and examined in anatomical detail over and over again. Although a person does indeed have a biological basis and can, in part, be explained in organic terms, this is only a small part of understanding the person in health care research. Care ought to entail viewing the person as a whole, psychological and social factors being regarded as just as influential as the biological factors. So, how far can persons be researched scientifically? Duffy (1985) remarks that there is an overemphasis in nursing research upon a scientific and quantitative approach. Nevertheless, she also acknowledges that nursing research ought to rely both upon both the true experiment, which emphasises the quantitative approach by seeking to identify truths, by isolating significant variables and controlling for intervening variables; and upon grounded theory which emphasises the qualitative approach, attemps to search for meaning, takes into account the social and environmental factors and treats its participants as subjects rather than objects. In other words, Duffy is advocating the usefulness of both positivism and a phenomenological perspective for health care research.

Positivistic research is a scientific approach to extending knowledge and generalising about the findings. The natural sciences are amenable to positivistic research because their subject matter can be broken down into its parts and studied under laboratory conditions. Research that is based on the so-called positivistic, scientific or true experimental basis, is seen to rest upon objective investigation and analysis based upon rational argument and an observation of the facts (Harris, 1979). The goal is to establish general laws about some phenomenon, regardless of the setting. To achieve this goal, positivistic methodology isolates and reduces variables (the person would be reduced to the status of object), such variables are then observed, quantified and analysed (can the personhood feature of thought, for example, be observed and measured?) Positivistic research is particularly concerned to establish causal laws or cause-and-effect relationships. For example the generalisation that smoking can cause cancer. But we also know that cancer is not necessarily caused by smoking and that not all people who are heavy smokers contract cancer. The development of generalised laws, suggesting certain knowledge, facts or truths that are applicable in all cases, is fallacious when applied to persons (Mischler, 1979).

To expect to be able to study the person outside of his/her natural setting and in a laboratory is a misguided practice and ignores the influence of the social context, relationships and experience. To quantify and statistically analyse the person gives a meaningless numerical description rather than any clear understanding and meaningful interpretation. To assume that a person can be understood by observation, negates the presence and influence of cognitive processes like thoughts, feelings, intentions, purposes, motivations, emotions, perceptions and experiences. People cannot be treated as things and cannot be generalised about, particularly in areas of health, well-being and illness. Although there are similarities between people that can be identified, the individual differences remain. For example, there could be ten people in a hospital ward, all with coronary heart disease, but each of those ten people would think, feel and react differently to this experience which necessarily includes biological, psychological and social aspects. It seems essential to avoid a purely positivistic approach in certain areas of health care research. Further, it substantiates the claim to integrate the social sciences and humanities into the health carers' curriculum and supports a more qualitative approach towards health care research.

A **phenomenological** perspective emphasises the centrality of how the individual person interacts in a social world of everday commonsense experience. Health care research, adopting this perspective, studies the person within their social context rather than in isolation and attempts to understand the meaning of their experiences. Grounded theory, which attempts to generate theory through the understanding of the person's own perception and interpretation of experience, underpins the phenomenological approach to research (Glaser and Strauss, 1967). It is a highly qualitative, descriptive and exploratory approach which is useful to the human science domains. It does not seek one truth for the purposes of explanation but recognises that many different but equal truths may be appropriate (Mischler, 1979). Because people perceive the world in a unique, idiosyncratic and constantly changing way, there may be any number of different ways of understanding persons and their experiences in a social world. Typical research questions that may be appropriate for a phenomenological approach include: what is it like to be a nurse/radiographer/occupational therapist? What is your conception of health care? What was your experience of pain like?

There are problems involved in carrying out highly qualitative research, and caution is necessary in selecting a method for data collection that matches the choice of study and the questions asked. Choosing methods depends upon what one wishes to know, what the expected outcome of the research will be, the constraints of the setting and, to a lesser extent, the resources available. In most cases, proving an hypothesis or answering a research question is difficult from a phenomenological basis; it is not like the highly quantifiable scientific investigations whose subject matter is open to reduction, observation, manipulation, objectivity and measurement. A theory will not necessarily be developed through a phenomenological perspective; the study will probably remain exploratory by its very nature and contribute, not in terms of any direct answer, but in terms of a clearer understanding. As James (1977) remarks, qualitative research "provides perspective, insight and understandable description."

SUMMARY

When talking about health care research, the emphasis is usually upon adding to existing knowledge and upon the understanding of such issues as health, illness, treatment and care. Central to these issues is the concept of the person.

A quantitative, scientific and positivistic approach is more appropriate if the aim of the research is to measure particular variables, specific biological/physical aspects of the individual, or certain objective facts about hospitals, clinics and numbers of patients, may be to discover the age-range and sex of recognised AIDS patients in a particular location. This kind of objective data allows for statistical analysis. A qualitative and phenomenological approach is more appropriate for subjective data that cannot be measured or clearly observed; rather it requires inference, assessment, interpretation and emphasis upon meaning and understanding. Examples may be nurses' attitudes towards smoking and health professionals' conceptions of care. The individual differences in attitudes and conceptions cannot be adequately reflected through numbers; it is essential to take into account the meaning and use of language and the subjective experience of the individual in terms of his/her unique ways of perceiving.

Much of the research in the area of health care is of a qualitative nature; hence, in later sections, the methods suitable for collecting qualitative information are reviewed.

DISCUSSION POINTS

1. Think of a research topic that would best be suited to a positivistic approach and one which would be more appropriated for a phenomenological approach.

2. Why is it difficult to generalise the findings deriving from research concerning persons?

3. What aspects of the person could be studied in a laboratory setting?

4. Ought research findings be thought of as new knowledge and facts, or as beliefs?

USEFUL READING

Anderson, R.J., Hughes, J. A. and Sharrock, W.W. (1986). *Philosophy and the Human Sciences,* Croom Helm, London

Duffy, M.E. (1985). Designing nursing research: the qualitative/quantitative debate. *J. Adv. Nurs.* **10**, 225–232

Field, P.A. and Morse, J.M. (1985). *Nursing Research: The Application of Qualitative Research*, Croom Helm, London

Glaser, B.G. and Strauss, A.L. (1967). *The Discovery of Grounded Theory: Strategies for Qualitative Research,* New York

Harris, M. (1979). *Research Strategies and the Structure of Science,* New York

Hughes, J. (1990). *The Philosophy of Social Research,* 2nd edn. Longman, New York

Mischler, E. (1979). Meaning in context: Is there any other kind? Harvard Educ. Rev., **49**, 119

Polit, D.F. and Hungler, B.F. (1987). *Nursing Research: Principles and Methods*, Lippincott – Harper Row, London

Chapter 2

Types of research

Most nursing research to date has been empirical. Nevertheless, it is possible to apply historical and philosophical/theoretical research to the health care domain.

Historical

In this form of research, documents and reports are analysed by the researcher who then relates them to events, developments or individuals who are central to the contents of the documents and reports, for example, the Mental Health Act specifically concerns psychiatric health professionals, legal professionals and mentally ill patients. The historical researcher will use either primary sources of information, i.e. original documents, such as Nursing Acts or Project 2000, or secondary sources of information, i.e. summaries, often presented in texts or journals such as the Nursing Times.

Philosophical/theoretical

In this form of research, the tools of logic and reason are used to extend knowledge. Analysis occurs with words, their meaning, use and effect. The relevance of philosophical research could enhance a clearer understanding for the health professional in relation to the knowledge they use and how they apply it. For example, philosophical analysis could be carried out on the concept of care in order to determine what form of knowledge base is most appropriate for its understanding in professional practice. Few health professionals, however, have used this form of research, although Schrock (1977) did attempt some analysis.

Empirical

The empirical researcher obtains his/her information from the subjects in the field. Various choices of research design are available, such as descriptive, experimental or action research. The choice depends upon the question or hypothesis that the researcher wishes to study. Methods of enquiry can be either qualitative and/or quantitative.

Descriptive research, which includes the survey method, involves large numbers of subjects and, as its name implies, seeks to describe the information obtained.

Experimental research is required where cause-and-effect relationships between two variables are looked for, and where predictions and generalisations are the aim. In experimental research, the variables are manipulated and not just described.

Action research is appropriate for qualitative studies dealing with highly evaluative, complex and non-predictable variables, like attitudes or conceptions. One example of action research is the case study.

Given that empirical research takes its principles from the scientific domain, it is useful to consider briefly some of the philosophical assumptions that underpin research.

The major assumptions are that scientific endeavours should be systematic, controlled, concerned to establish cause-and-effect relationships and to formulate generalised laws and theories in order that predictions can be made. For example, the particular observation that the sun has risen every morning leads to the generalised theory that the sun will always rise in the morning. This kind of claim is more acceptable within the natural sciences than the social and human sciences, because it is not the case that an individual will always respond in a particular way to a particular situation. However, some philosophers of science support the idea that knowledge, truth and certainty are not clear-cut issues. Popper (1968), for instance, claimed that laws and theories must remain hypothetical since they can always be superceded by better ones which would approximate more accurately towards the truth. Knowledge can be viewed as relative. For example, it was once 'known' that the world was flat. New information revised this claim to say that the world was, in fact, round. In this sense, science, knowledge and fact have to be attributed with a subjective element and seen also to involve individual beliefs and preferences for one competing theory over another. Therefore, if research takes its principles from science, then research also must be viewed as not totally value free, rational and objective.

DISCUSSION POINTS

1. Think of a research topic where you as the researcher could utilise primary sources of information.

2. What would be an appropriate health related research topic for theoretical analysis?

3. Are theories of nursing knowledge or belief?

USEFUL READING

Chalmers, A.F. (1978). *What is this Thing Called Science?* Oxford University Press

Cohen, L. and Manion, L. (1980). *Research Methods in Education*, Croom Helm, London

Macleod-Clark, J. and Hockey, L. (1979). *Research for Nursing*, A Guide for the Enquiring Nurse, H.M. and M., London

Chapter 3

The ethical issues of research

A major rule in any kind of applied research is 'respect for persons'. This involves a concern for their welfare and respect for the respondents' wishes (Harris 1985). Further, health care research may involve studying, in detail, the work of individual doctors, nurses, social workers and other health professionals. Moral problems are involved in situations where care may be substandard or deficient, or where there are inadequate resources. A study to investigate a clinical unit may indicate that additional nursing staff are required. Another investigation may show that the lack of Ethics in the curricula of the health professions affects how the health professional copes with particular situations or makes decisions vital to the patient experiencing care. The researcher will have to deal with the moral problems involved in these findings, and this raises the question of the role of the researcher.

Much of the literature in the field of moral aspects of research deals with the rights of the patient. Clark and Robinson (1989) suggest that care, consent and confidentiality are central to the moral concerns and rights of the patient involved in health research. It is also the case that those individuals carrying out the research may have their own moral problems to deal with. As Clark and Robinson note, health care researchers should be aware, not only of the patient's rights, but also of their own professional codes and committees.

What ought to be done if a research assistant is providing inaccurate results by fiddling or fixing the numbers, or altering statements made by respondents?

What happens if a researcher is not suited to studying the psychological impact of some forms of treatment, for example, a health professional who, on a personal level, objects to the use of electroconvulsive therapy?

Who should be informed if a regional health research project identifies one particular hospital as showing a bad record regarding infection and disease?

If medical research and nursing research suggest a conflict in relation to the well-being of the patient, what ought to be done?

Researchers cannot detach themselves from the results of their studies. Those health professionals who are involved in research must take responsibility for the moral implications of the research process, how it is carried out and the results.

How are the priorities for funding health care research established? A basic conflict is between the need to find out basic research, which might lead to fundamental changes in our understanding of disease, and research identifying more appropriate forms of health care. If funding is limited, difficult choices have to be made, for example, ought quality assurance to be given priority over patients' well-being, or is dementia in the elderly less or more of a priority than research focussing upon *in vitro* fertilisation?

Ethical committees and codes of practice are designed to aid in the decision-making processes underlying health care research. They are set up to monitor research proposals and to safeguard both the patient and the researcher. Members of ethical committees ought to have an education in professional ethics and, therefore, be well informed of the ethical codes for research which must be universally applicable across the health profession. Health care is best delivered through a team approach; hence, ethical codes ought not to be exclusive to one profession, i.e. the medical doctors.

Sheehan (1985) suggests that nursing practice is concerned to enhance professional knowledge whilst retaining a professional ethic. Although research is necessary to the development of knowledge and understanding in the health care domain, it must also emphasise the need to pursue patient care and the protection of the patient's rights. To achieve the latter, constant reflection and critical analysis of health care practice must rest upon moral integrity. According to Faulder (1985), an excessive number of patients are being used in clinical trials without their knowledge or consent. The doctors performing these trials, justify this action by claiming 1) that the patients do not understand the scientific reasons underlying the study and 2)that patients would lose their confidence in doctors if they were informed that clinical trials were being carried out because it suggests that the doctors do not know the best forms of treatment. The kind of violation of human rights implicit within this type of experimental research does not reflect professional moral integrity. It not only generates negative physical, psychological and emotional effects on those involved, but may also foster a general resistance to and lack of trust in research and researchers.

Shrock (1984) points out that nursing research involves delving into the private activities and experiences of a broad spectrum of people. This raises a great many moral issues and ethical concerns. The International Council of Nurses *Guidelines for Nursing Research Development* (1985) recognises these moral issues and

The ethical issues of research

claims. Since much of nursing research involves persons, "it is necessary the dignity, human rights and welfare of the subjects be considered and protected adequately according to the ethical principles of the profession." Health practitioners ought to act as responsible professionals between the demands of the researcher and the needs and rights of the patient in order to ensure against any kind of abuse. Health professionals should be able to ask appropriate questions of researchers and be able to critically consider the research proposals prior to agreeing to participate in any research.

Clark and Robinson (1989) have drawn up an exceptionally useful list of questions that health professionals should consider in detail:

i) Is the researcher who is proposing to undertake the study sufficiently qualified and experienced?

ii) Can the proposed study be justified. In other words, has such a study been carried out previously and is there a need for an additional study?

iii) Is the research question worthwhile trying to answer?

iv) Has the research proposal been designed to address the research question?

v) How carefully has the research proposal been designed?
vi) Has an ethical committee approved the research?
vii) Are patients, their families or health professionals likely to be put at risk in any way or inconvenienced by the research?
viii) How are the findings going to be used, and by whom?
ix) Has the researcher addressed the issues of privacy, confidentiality and anonymity?
x) Is consent to participate in the research required and, if so, how will this be obtained and recorded?
xi) Are the sources to fund the research adequate?

DISCUSSION POINTS

1. Can you think of an health care research proposal which would not show respect for persons?

2. What sort of research proposal would infringe upon a patient's rights?

3. Try to think of potential conflicts between the demands of science and the demands of ethics which could affect the design of the research.

USEFUL READING

Clark, E. and Robinson K.M. (1989). *Nursing Research: Ethics and Methods, Module 6,* South Bank Polytechnic, London

Downie, R.S. and Calman, K.C. (1987). *Healthy Respect: Ethics in Health Care,* Faber and Faber

Faulder, C. (1985). *Whose Body Is It? The Troubling Issue of Informed Consent,* Virago

Harris, J. (1985). *The Value of Life,* Routledge and Kegan Paul

Henry, I.C. and Pashley, G. (1990). *Health Ethics,*Health and Nursing Studies for Diploma and Undergraduate Students, Quay Publishing, Lancaster

Hockey, L. (1985). *Nursing Research: Mistakes and Misconceptions,* Churchill Livingstone

Schrock, R. (1984). Moral issues in nursing research, *The Research Process in Nursing,* Cormack, D.F.S. (ed.), Blackwell

Sheehan, J. (1985). Ethical considerations in nursing practice, *J. Adv. Nurs.,* **10,** 331–336

Chapter 4

Preparation and design for completing research

The raw material of research is not pieces of information but ideas; ideas which can be tested, measured, examined, assessed or interpreted by collecting data. The data can reveal whether the initial idea was valid or inadequate.

In any kind of research, there are particular stages through which to proceed. First, identify and define the problem on the basis of reading primary and secondary sources, for example, textbooks, research articles and reports. This initial stage is crucial in the whole process, for the [...] of the remaining stages of the research depe[...] thoroughly the problem has been th[...]nning. Ideas take shape a[...]nowledge; hence, the [...]re likely the idea [...] be original, [...] of a review [...]ve written and discover[...] it is essential to read as widel[...] and how others have approached the same kind of topic. As the researcher's knowledge broadens, he/she begins to formulate hypotheses or research questions which define the boundaries of the problem more precisely. The reading should not be restrictive and narrow because important contributions to research have resulted from the cross-fertilisation of disciplines and subject matter. However, it is important also that, by the time the researcher is ready to commence any data collection or writing up of the literature, he/she should have identified the priorities, been selective and focussed on particular theoretical knowledge and research findings that are pertinent to the nature of the intended research.

Second, having defined the precise field of the research, it is necessary to decide how best to collect the information, from whom this information is to be obtained and to know how much time and resources are available to complete this task. Choosing the research methodology is very much influenced by the nature of the research and the preferences of the researcher. For example, if a researcher is concerned with describing the activities and conversations of, say, individual professionals or patients, a group of professionals, or children in hospital, then his/her methodology may very much depend upon the skills of observation and recording data. If a researcher is more concerned with understanding the meaning that a health professional attaches to the concept of care, then an in-depth and open-ended interview may be more appropriate. In effect, the researcher has to decide upon the relative advantages and disadvantages of the chosen research methods over and above others which might have been suitable.

The subjects of an investigation are the people who are involved in the study and who will provide the information on which the investigation is based. Often a piece of research is planned with a certain kind of individual in mind. It may relate to a group of professionals in a particular hospital or community, a group of persons experiencing health care either in hospital or the community, or it may be children or adults of a particular age range and with a particular illness or disease. Most researchers are well-advised to choose subjects of a type with which they are familiar. The question of the number of subjects to be involved in the sample is determined, to a large extent, by the nature of the research, resources available and choice of methodology. For example, a questionnaire is easily distributed to a large number of subjects but it may not be appropriate for the kind of data the researcher wishes to collect, nor may the researcher have the funds to post a large number of questionnaires with prepaid envelopes for their return upon completion.

Having collected the data, the next stage in the research process is deciding what to do with the results. The analysis of the data is greatly influenced by the research methodology, for instance, if the data is numerical, like age and sex of the subjects, then it is more amenable to statistical analysis. If the information is qualitative, say, interview transcripts, then it has to be interpreted, perhaps through a procedure of coding and classifying it in some way. The final stage involved in the research process is that of writing up the findings and discussing them in relation to the hypotheses or research questions, the theoretical basis of the research and previous research carried out.

When the general plan of an investigation is complete, it is wise to try it out on a small scale. This is the **pilot study** and serves to provide the researcher with an opportunity to practice adminstering tests or interviewing skills. It may bring to light weaknesses in methodology so that amendments can be made prior to the actual research, for example, an extra question may be written into the interview schedule.

The following example serves to illustrate how the stages of a research process can be applied:

Problem/bright idea – it seems to be the case that nurses act as counsellors but are not confident in the role of counsellor. It would be interesting to find out what the nurses themselves think.

Tentative hypotheses/research questions:

1. It will be found that nurses are not clear about what is meant by the term 'counselling'.

2. It will be evident that the nurse perceives his/her role as incorporating that of a counsellor.

3. There will be support for the idea that nurses should receive more social skills training and counselling techniques in their professional education.

The problem could be more clearly defined through a theoretical literature review, for example, by looking at the history of counselling, the different theories and therapies in counselling, and through a review of previous research, preferably relating to the nurse/patient relationship, family/nurse relationship or counselling relationship between health professionals.

Since the aim is to identify how nurses conceive of counselling, a qualitative approach to methodology is required. An interview will allow the researcher to ask nurses about their views and ideas regarding counselling. The interview questions might include, "What does the term 'counselling' mean to you?" "Do you see yourself as a counsellor?" and "Should more emphasis be placed upon counselling skills in your professional education?" Interviews can generate a great deal of information for interpretation; therefore, small numbers will be involved in the sample, say, 20–40 respondents. Included in this sample, will be a mixture of male and female qualified general and psychiatric nurses, in order to identify whether sex and the type of nurse, influences conceptions

The interview schedule which has been developed needs to be tried out with, perhaps, five nurses, in order to determine whether any questions need to be changed, omitted, or added. Once the pilot study has been carried out and the changes made, the main study of all the subjects involved in the sample can take place. Interviews will be tape-recorded and subsequently transcribed.

Preparation and design for completing research

The interview transcriptions then need to be analysed and interpreted in order to identify the similarities and differences in conceptions between the groups of respondents. The discussion of the results reveals that nurses could not explain clearly what the term counselling meant, but they felt it was something they did in their role as a nurse (so research questions 1 and 2 are supported). A number of nurses are found to prefer a humanistic approach. A large number of respondents think that counselling skills should form an important part of professional education (so research question 3 was supported). The following diagram serves to show how the stages of a research project link to its presentation

STAGES IN A RESEARCH PROJECT	FORMAL PRESENTATION OF, A MASTERS DISSERTATION OR PhD
Identifying and precisely defining the problem	Chapter 1 Literature review
Reading previous research on relevant topics	Chapter 2 Research review
Deciding on techniques to be used for collecting and analysing data Selecting and defining the sample Collecting the data	Chapter 3 Design and Procedure of study (incorporating research methodology, pilot study and main study
Processing, analysing and interpreting results	Chapter 4 Analysis of Results
Writing up the report	Chapter 5 Discussion of results

DISCUSSION POINTS

1. How important is it to read other theorists and researchers work?

2. Why is the research methodology influenced by the nature of the research?

3. How important is the pilot study and what is its main purpose?

4. Why must the form of data analysis match the type of research?

USEFUL READING

Cohen, L. and Manion, L. (1980). *Research Methods in Education*, Croom Helm

Howard, K. and Sharp, J. A. (1983). *The Management of a Student Research Project*, Gower Publishing

Chapter 5

The questionnaire

According to Nesbit and Entwistle (1970), the questionnaire is similar to an interview on paper; therefore, just as much care is essential in the construction of questions and choice of words. The questionnaire is impersonal; there is no face-to-face interaction with the researcher which would allow him/her to explain the purpose, procedure and possible ambiguities or misunderstandings. For this reason, it is important that a questionnaire comprises the same features as a 'good law', and that it is:

> "....clear, unambiguous and uniformly workable. Its design must minimise potential errors from respondents... and coders. And since people's participation in surveys is voluntary, a questionnaire has to help in engaging their interest, encouraging their co-operation and eliciting answers as close as possible to the truth." (Davidson, 1970)

The questionnaire allows the researcher to collect information from a small or large number of people, either on a local level or on a national level. If the research is to involve, say, student nurses in all the schools and colleges of nursing throughout England and Wales, or all qualified occupational therapists with a particular health authority, then a postal-type questionnaire would be more economical in terms of cost, time and labour. Further, the same questionnaire could be distributed to a large number of individuals and information collected in a uniform and structured way (Cohen and Manion, 1980). These are the main advantages of the questionnaire. However, there is another advantage which could also count as a disadvantage. The questionnaire is impersonal, and this is a weakness in the sense that any form of interpersonal contact between the researcher and the respondent is either non-existent or negligible. This feature could be viewed as an advantage in that it preserves the anonymity of the respondent; the respondent need not be seen, need not reveal his/her name and can complete the questionnaire in private.

The main disadvantage of the questionnaire is the fact that respondents are limited in expanding upon their views, ideas, feelings and reasons for choosing the answer they did, because only a fixed set of alternative choices are presented. In general format, all questionnaires are basically the same; consisting of a series of items describing, attitudes, feelings or reactions to everyday situations like work, illness, pain stress. The respondent is asked to indicate whether any of the items are typical of him/her. The answers are usually restricted to: *Yes/No, True/False, Always/Never/Sometimes, Agree/Don't know/Disagree.* Further disadvantages lie with the fact that the researcher is not provided with the opportunity to probe for more detail, and is unavailable to explain any misunderstandings that may arise because the questions are fixed and structured. For this reason, it is of paramount importance that the construction and design of the questionnaire is clear, unambiguous and asks the kind of questions which will generate the precise information that the researcher seeks, and which will encourage respondents to freely provide the necessary answers.

There is a general belief that the rate of return of completed questionnaires is not always encouraging. Nesbit and Entwistle remark that a response rate of less than 70 percent implies the findings will lack validity for general application. It is interpreted that one out of three respondents will have chosen not to complete and return the questionnaire, and that this is too large a proportion of the sample to disregard. It is important that the researcher makes some attempt to discover the reason for this. Cohen and Manion (1980) suggest that a low rate of response to a questionnaire is not a general pattern and that if it is designed appropriately the response rate can be very good. To secure a good response, certain criteria must be met that will foster the perception of the questionnaire by the respondent as worthwhile, attractively presented and straightforward to complete and return. In order to facilitate the preparation of a 'good' questionnaire, the researcher should have:

1. Precisely defined the nature and extent of the research problem,

2. Clearly identified the sample of subjects or population at whom the questionnaire is to be directed

3. Begun to frame the questions around the precise research problem and the sample subjects.

The questions need to be constructed so as to ensure that the responses will answer the research problem and the related hypotheses. It is essential that the wording and arrangement of the questions are well thought out and construed. The questionnaire is best used for relatively simple and factual enquiries. It should begin with simple, factual questions in order to encourage respondents. Complex questions are more appropriately placed in the middle of the questionnaire and they should be introduced gradually. It is important to note that complex questions may be answered superficially by respondents, especially if they are perceived as threatening, too difficult or too invasive of privacy. Some respondents may answer the questions in terms of how they anticipate the researcher wants them to answer; others may refuse to answer certain types of questions. It is better to leave open-ended questions until the close of the questionnaire. This allows the respondent to comment on what he/she perceives to be important issues, and perhaps to identify areas that have not been covered but ought to be considered. These points emphasise that the careful wording and arrangement of questions is of central importance. Questionnaires rely on words, and it is necessary to be aware that the same words can mean different things to different people; there is much ambiguity in the meaning and use of language. For example, what one respondent means by 'patient care', 'psychological therapy' or 'counselling the patient and family' may not be the same as the meaning attached to these same terms and phrases by another.

Simplicity, clarity and brevity are essential criteria of a 'good' questionnaire. Constructing and designing a functional questionnaire implies that certain types of questions and words are avoided:

1. Avoid leading questions which tend to suggest what the answer should be, for example, "Do you

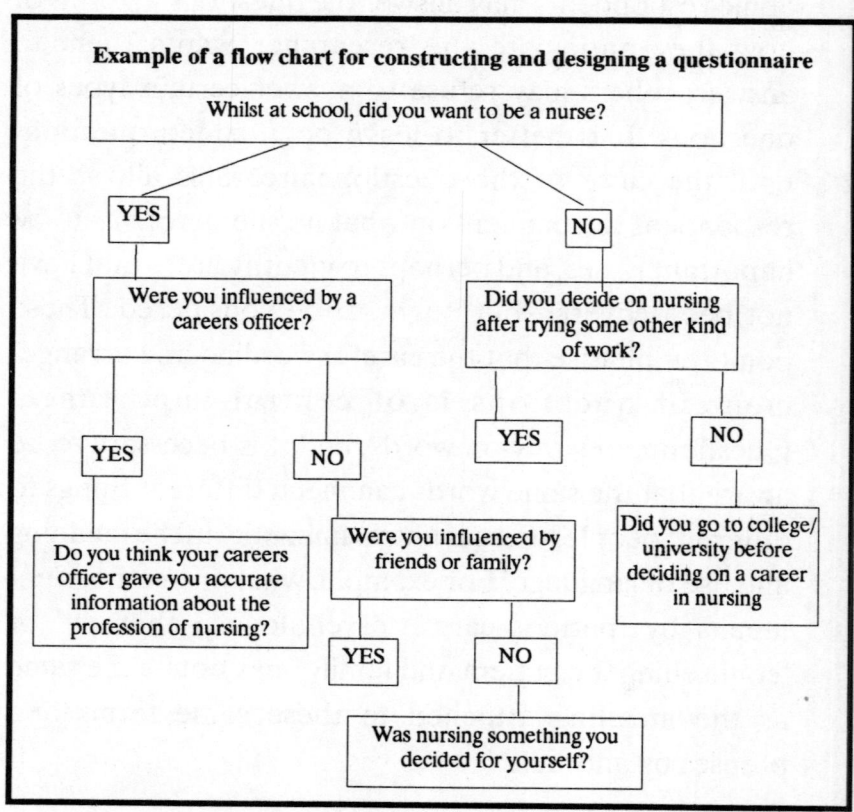

think nurse education should be research-led or simply left to commonsense and trial and error?"

2. Avoid complex, abstract and open-ended questions (although an open-ended question is sometimes useful at the end of the questionnaire), for example, "What phenomenological features of the person are central to understanding health and illness behaviour?

3. Avoid irritating questions, such as, "Have you ever attended a post-basic course of any kind in your entire professional career as a nurse?"

4. Avoid negative questions, for example, "How strongly do you feel that no nurse who has not been qualified for more than two years, should counsel a terminally ill patient and his/her family?"

5. Avoid loaded words which are usually emotionally coloured, for example, Nazis, motherly, intelligent.

A flow chart can be useful in planning the sequence of questions and enables the researcher to anticipate the type and range of responses that the questions may elicit.

If a questionnaire is being posted to the subjects or being distributed to the respondents without the researcher having the opportunity to discuss and explain the research, then it is essential that a covering letter accompanies the questionnaires. Such a letter plays an important role in the sense that it can be used to persuade the subjects to participate. It should explain the purpose of the research, emphasise the importance of the information which the respondents could provide, verify that the information will be treated as confidential and close with a sentence that encourages a response. Response rates can also be improved if, enclosed with the letter is a prepaid and pre-addressed envelope for the return of the questionnaire. It is important that the questionnaire appears attractive, is well laid out and easy to complete, with clear instructions on how to answer the questions.

Completed and returned questionnaires provide information which requires classification and coding for the purposes of analysis and interpretation. The responses can be coded in order to transform them into numerical data, for example, **YES** could be coded as **1**, and **NO** could be coded as 2. It is useful if the questionnaire is initially designed to take into account its eventual analysis and, therefore, to construct questions and alternative answers that facilitate the procedure of precoding possible answers. In other words, the researcher should know in advance how the yes/no, agree/don't know/disagree responses are going to be coded and numerically represented. Although this potential numerical data can provide useful information, it must be interpreted with care because a limited set of alternative answers may force the respondent into an uneasy and inaccurate choice. The interpretation of information generated by the questionnaire can often profitably be considered alongside other research methodology, for example, the interview.

DISCUSSION POINTS

1. Think about how you would pilot a questionnaire.

2. Construct a flow diagram to help with the construction of questions that you would like answered.

USEFUL READING

Cohen, L. and Manion, L. (1980). *Research Methods in Education*, Croom Helm

Field, P.A. and Morse, J.M. (1985). *Nursing Research: The Application of Qualitative Research*, Croom Helm

Marsh, C. (1983). *The Survey Method*, George Allen and Unwin

Nesbit, J.D. and Entwistle, N.J. (1970). *Educational Research Methods*, University of London Press

Oppenheim, A.N. (1966). *Questionnaire Design and Attitude Measurement*, Heinemann

Skevington, S. (ed.) (1984). *Understanding Nurses: The Social Psychology of Nursing*, Wiley & Son

Chapter 6

The interview

As a research technique, the interview, like the questionnaire, is considered to be one of the survey methods. Interviews can be rigid or flexible and can be used for a variety of purposes, for example: to explore peoples' attitudes, opinions or conceptions; to draw inferences about peoples' behaviour; or to attempt some understanding of peoples' emotional reactions, e.g. the feelings associated with learning that you have cancer or multiple sclerosis.

There are several different types of interview which can be used for a variety of purposes; the choice is determined by the nature of the research and the questions or hypotheses that are being examined.

The formal or **structured** interview is when the questions asked are set or fixed and responses are easily recorded, classified and coded. This type of interview is quite similar to the questionnaire. Cohen and Manion (1980) remark that the content and the procedures of the structured interview are determined in advance and that this format prevents the interviewer from making modifications to the sequence or wording of the questions.

The **less formal** or **semistructured** interview allows the researcher to modify the sequence of question to some degree, to slightly change the wording and to insert an occasional additional question or to explain the questions if necessary.

The **informal, unstructured** or **open-ended** interview has the qualities of freedom and flexibility. The researcher can raise a number of key issues in a far more conversational style. The open-ended interview, in particular, is essentially exploratory in the sense that the researcher is attempting to encourage people to reveal and reflect upon specific issues. It is ideal for more complex, abstract and controversial subjects.

According to Nesbit and Entwistle (1970), the research interview is a live, direct and verbal method of collecting information; a two-person conversation initiated by the interviewer for the specific purpose of obtaining answers can be organised and used to give an overall picture relevant to the objectives of the research.

The remainder of this section is specifically concerned with the open-ended interview because it generates the kind of information central to health care research, which needs to be qualitatively interpreted in order to assess meaning and understanding (Finch 1985). As James (1977) remarks, qualitative research

The interview

"provides perspective, insight and understandable description."

The open-ended interview allows a more personal approach to be adopted and, because of its flexibility and adaptability, facilitates freedom on the part of the interviewer and respondent. This type of interview encourages rapport, provides the opportunity for probing and places minimum restraint on the respondent's answers and expressions (Cohen and Manion 1980). However, there are a number of problems and disadvantages associated with the interview technique:

1. The number of subjects involved in the research is restricted because face-to-face interview situations are time consuming, require organisation in terms of date, time and appropriate location, and yield a large amount of rich information which needs interpreting.

2. Numerous sources of error prevail: errors relating to the research tool itself, the coding and misinterpretation of responses, the actual sample of subjects and the interviewer him/herself.

Burgess (1985) remarks on the position of the interviewer and suggests that, where the interviewer and respondent are unknown to each other and where they have different occupations, the interviewer is at an advantage in the sense that he/she can set and manage the discussion. Burgess goes on to claim that the situation becomes more complex when the interviewer is asking questions of his/her peers; the advantage of possessing superior knowledge or techniques is lost. Equally, the respondent can make assumptions that certain things do not need to be explained and, as a result, gaps can appear in the information. The important point here is that peers should be aware that they may share a common knowledge but ought not to take this for granted. The onus lies with the interviewer to ask the respondent to expand on particular comments.

The sources of error mentioned can be minimised to some extent, if subjectivity and bias on the part of the interviewer are reduced. Cohen and Manion suggest the following ways in which subjectivity and bias can be lessened:

1. Careful formulation of questions so that the meaning is precise,

2. Thorough training in interviewing skills,

3. Probability sampling (i.e. where the type of re-

spondent is selected),

4. Matching interviewer characteristics with those of the sample being interviewed.

A final comment concerning the interview involves the use of tape recordings. This method of recording information is held to be more advantageous than note taking because the latter task frequently results in a lack of continuity in the social interaction. Burgess remarks that note taking does not result in detailed material as it is impossible to record fully in note form, the replies which respondents verbalise. She comments also, that note taking is time consuming given the amount of information, and that the procedure makes the interview more formal and stilted. Her conclusions are that tape recordings prove invaluable for keeping a full and accurate record of the discussion. There are problems associated with taping responses. For example, the transcription can often result in the oversimplification of complex human, speech, transforming it into smooth prose (Henry 1985). A related problem is that of content analysis, i.e. interpreting the transcripts on the basis of word counts. The underlying rationale is that categories are constructed, words are extracted from the transcripts and then, if they fit the categories, they are counted as such. The danger with this approach is one of assuming that words used by all of the respondents have the same meaning. For this reason it is important that the interviewer probes in sufficient depth so that he/she can determine the respondent's precise meaning.

Designing and constructing an interview schedule needs the same care as planning a questionnaire. The first step is the formulation of the aims and objectives of the research; this initially derives from 'bright ideas' that are subsequently supported by, and grounded in, theoretical knowledge, and an awareness of previous and similar research carried out. The second step is to think about the preparation of the interview schedule; how structured or unstructured it should be, to ensure that the questions are clear, unambiguous and will generate the kind of information required to support or invalidate the research questions/hypotheses. It is sensible to start with simple questions for the purposes of establishing some kind of rapport through an easy exchange of conversation. More complex or personal questions need to be worked in gradually. A sequential flow of questions can often facilitate the flow and ease of the interaction between the interviewer and respondent, but this depends upon the content of the responses.

The wording of the questions is also important. It is better to avoid jargon and necessary to remember that the interviewer is at an advantage in terms of familiarity with the nature of the research and the interview questions. All subjects in the sample should be able to understand the words used. Consideration should be given to the sample of subjects who are selected as being representative of a particular population. For example, a question about 'nursing models' may well be appropriate for nurses but could be meaningless for radiographers or speech therapists. Questions which are biased in the sense of encouring a 'yes' response with supportive reasons should also be avoided, for example, "Don't you agree that Project 2000 is an innovative and essential development for the nursing profession?"

When the interviewing is complete, the researcher has to interpret the responses. All the key phrases which the respondents have mentioned could be underlined, but this may lead to misinterpretation by the interviewer. The meaning attached to the phrase "assessment of care" may vary with each respondent. The meaning and use of language is social, ambiguous, subjective and has to be understood in relation to the sentence context in which the phrase occurs, and to the social context in which it is said. This links to a further potential problem for the researcher. He/she must acknowledge that what a respondent says may not accurately reflect what goes on in practice. For example, a psychiatric nurse may claim that punishment for a mentally ill person is absolutely inappropriate or even wrong, and yet support seclusion or withdrawal of privileges as part of a treatment programme. The question arises, "are seclusion and withdrawal of privileges forms of treatment or punishment?" Nevertheless, the researcher generally looks for patterns in the interview transcripts and has to make some attempt at understanding the contents. Responses may be coded before or after the interview for the purposes of analysis and/or interpretation; much depends upon the nature of the research, the type of interview used and the questions asked.

As with the questionnaire, it is essential that a pilot study is carried out, regardless of whether the interview is of the formal, less formal or open-ended type. This procedure will give the researcher the invaluable opportunity to test whether or not the type of interview and the sequence and wording are appropriate, whether any questions need deleting, amending or adding, and which particular questions need probing for more detail by the interviewer. During the pilot run, the interview can be tape recorded and subsequently listened to and transcribed. This will highlight the style of the interaction and ease the task of identifying any flaws in the whole procedure.

DISCUSSION POINTS

1. Summarise the main advantages and disadvantages of the open-ended interview.

2. For what type of research would you use the formal interview, the less formal interview and the open-ended interview?

3. What would you need to consider before deciding whether to use a questionnaire or a type of interview?

USEFUL READING

Burgess, R.G. (1985). *Issues in Educational Research*, Falmer Press

Cohen, L. and Manion, L. (1980). *Research Methods in Education*, Croom Helm

Finch, J. (1985). Social policy and education: problems and possibilities of using qualitative research, *Issues in Educational Research*, Burgess, R.G. (ed.) Falmer Press

James, J. (1977). Ethnography and social problems, *Street Ethnography*, Weppner, R.S. (ed.) Sage

Nesbit, J.D. and Entwistle, N.J. (1970). *Educational Research Methods*, University of London Press

Rose, S. *et al.*, (1985). Studying health and disease, *Open University Book 1, Course U205*, Open University Press

Skevington, S. (ed.) (1984). *Understanding Nurses: The Social Psychology of Nursing*, Wiley & Son

Chapter 7

Action research

Cohen and Manion (1980) and Kelly (1985) both acknowledge that giving a clear and comprehensive definition of action research is difficult. The terms 'action' and 'research' have separate meanings and are separate activities, and, when they are joined to represent a style of research within the social sciences, the definition becomes extremely complex. This issue is further complicated in that action research means different things to different people. Nevertheless, Hasley's definition (1972) is a useful starting point:

> *"action research is a small scale intervention in the functioning of the real world and a close examination of the effects of such intervention"*

Cohen and Manion identify four central features of action research:

1. It is **situational** in that the research is concerned with considering and solving a problem within the context in which it occurs.

2. There is a **collaborative** element due to the fact that team researchers and practitioners co-operate and work together on the problem.

3. It is **participatory** in the sense that the team researchers and practioners are directly and/or indirectly involved in the research and the solving of the problem.

4. There is an element of **self-evaluation**, implying that the researchers and practitioners are constantly making modifications on the basis of reviewing the situation and events taking place.

In effect, the prime aim is to improve practice and add to the practitioners functional knowledge base.

The scope of action research is wide; it can range from a health educator trying out novel ways of teaching health-related studies to his/her students, to a sophisticated study involving a team of research and health practitioners, or the organisational changes occurring in hospitals as a result of the implementation of quality assurance.

Action research is far more liberal in its interpretation of the scientific approach or method of applying research, essentially because it is focussing upon a particular problem in a particular social context. It is important that precise and functional knowledge and understanding be achieved as a result of action research, rather than findings which can be generalised.

Action could be suitably applied to the following examples:

1. Something which addresses itself to the personal functioning, interpersonal relationships and morale of particular health professionals (efficiency, motivation and well-being).

2. A concern for health professionals' functioning, effectiveness and efficiency (job analysis).

3. A focus on how innovation and change are implemented, for example Project 2000.

4. An interest in how to improve methods of continuous assessment.

The collaborative or co-operative element identified by Cohen and Manion, implying that teams of researchers and teams of professionals work together on problems occurring in particular social contexts, is now widely encouraged and emphasised. The knowledge, ideas and experience of both the researchers and the professional practitioners can be combined in order to solve a problem that has been identified and located in a particular situation. The problem is constantly monitored over a period of time and, through the use of a variety of research methods, for example question- naires, interviews, diaries, observations and case studies, information and feedback can be interpreted and utilised to introduce changes, modifications, redefinitions, or whatever has been highlighted as requiring adjustment or implementation. The findings and subsequent recommendations can be applied immediately; the changes which are shown to be necessary can be introduced without delay through group interaction and co-operation.

Action research is flexible, adaptable and relies essentially upon observation and behavioural information. In this sense, it is an empirical approach to research; information is collected, recorded, shared and discussed, evaluated and acted upon by both researchers and practitioners. However, there are several ciriticisms which can be levelled at action research. Because there is no attempt to isolate and study one or two particular factors or variables operating within a particular social context, it is held to lack the systematic rigour representative of 'true' experimental research. If health professionals and researchers are working on a collaborative basis, it is important to keep in mind that the two sets of professionals each have their own objectives, values, perceptions and experiences which could, potentially, foster a conflicting relationship. Although both parties share the same interest in solving a specific problem that is arising in a particular context, their respective viewpoints, levels of analysis, critical evaluation and interpretation may differ. This comes back to the original point, made at the beginning of this section, that action and research are separate activities. More specifically, health professionals may be more concerned with doing things and with action, whereas researchers may place more emphasis upon research values, such as precision, control, replication and generalisation. The potential for incompatibility and conflict between action and research can become a reality. However, the two must be synthesised through an identification of the problem and the context; a clear and comprehensive statement of the aims and objectives in solving the problem; an understanding, by all participants, of the implications of the project, and acceptance of each others' role within the project.

According to Kelly (1985), the specific methodology used in action research is seen to be less important than the approach taken towards action and research. Action research enhances knowledge and understanding because it deals with real situations and events, and recognises the complexity of interdependent factors and relationships. Action research should be a learning experience for all those individuals involved, and ought to facilitate professional development as a result of involvement and interaction.

Kelly puts forward the notion of **'simultaneous-integrated action research'.** This suggests that action and research can proceed concurrently, that they are mutually supportive. There should be no division of labour between practitioners and researchers for both have much to offer. Health professionals have the ideas, knowledge and potential to reflect upon their own experience in order to help in the identification of problems which, if changed in some way, can enhance professional practice. Researchers can point the direction for credible action, having taken into account, and discussed with the practitioners, their ideas and experiences in the planning stage, and assist in the evaluation process. Both practitioners and researchers need to be collaborative; both must be aware of the purposes and results of the project and both must be respectful of each others' ideas, knowledge, understanding and expertise.

According to Kelly, simultaneous-integrated action research can reduce the communication gap between practitioners and researchers through collaboration and shared involvement throughout the whole process. Practitioners can begin to value research, its methods and findings, particularly if the research has been carried out in the real world where professionals practice. Researchers are given the opportunity to become directly involved in social change, to extend knowledge and understanding, and to value the necessity of applying research in a natural and social setting in which practitioners operate.

DISCUSSION POINTS

1. Identify a particular problem, in either a hospital or community setting, where a team of health professionals/practitioners and researchers could collaborate and intervene in order to solve the problem.

USEFUL READING

Cohen, L. and Manion, L. (1980). *Methods in Education,* Croom Helm

Halsey, A.H. (ed.) (1972). *Educational Priority: Problems and Policies,* HMSO

Hulk, M. and Lennung, S. (1980). Towards a definition of action research, *J. Manage. Stud.* **17**, 2, 241–250

Kelly, A. (1985). Action research: what is it and what can it do?, *Issues in Educational Research,* Burgess, R.G. (ed.) Falmer Press

Powley, T. and Evans, D. (1979). Towards a methodology of action research, *J. Soc. Policy,* **8**, 27–46

Smith, G. (1982). Action Research 1968–81, Method of research or method of innovation?, *J. Commun. Educ.,* **1**, 31–46

Chapter 8

The case study

The case study, as its name implies, is a detailed study of a particular case or single individual. A case study is an approach whereby an individual is systematically observed and/or tested in great detail. Interestingly, the compiling of case studies is a major part of the education and experience of clinical psychologists. The end product is abundantly rich in detail and can be fascinating to read. In health care research, the focus may be upon the health or illness of an individual patient (Rose *et al*, 1985).

Case studies are in-depth inquiries about a single individual and may involve gathering data spanning his/her life experiences to date. Close observation of behaviour is also a central feature of the case study. This type of approach must have a definite purpose in order for it to be classed as research rather than simply an accumulation of information. For example, the purpose may be to understand why a patient is not recovering as quickly as expected by health professionals. Evans (1968) remarks that, although the case study may not be the kind of research that extends knowledge, it is valuable in the sense that it can identify more specific factors which might otherwise have been overlooked. There is a sense in which case studies can humanise the research and avoid the mere collection of a set of observations or facts. It emphasises the social world in which persons interact and experience reality.

Rose *et al,* remark that the case study is efficient at identifying odd, unusual or rare associations, but quite ineffective when it comes to recognising common associations, for example factors common to a number of individual patients with the same condition. Working with a single subject or patient does allow for detailed observations and experiments that simply cannot be conducted on a group of individuals. Neither can the findings derived from a single individual be applied to a similar group of individuals. Utilising the case study in health care research may be restrictive because the environmental contexts can be limited, for example a cancer patient may be confined to clinical settings, such as a hospital ward, hospice, outpatient department or clinic. Such environments may influence a patient's behaviour and, in turn, have an effect upon how the researcher observes and perceives the patient.

Skilbeck (1983) suggests, on one level, that the case study leads to the "perfection of observation and documentation." As stated earlier, observation is a central feature of the case study.

Cohen and Manion (1980) distinguish two types of observation:

Non-participant observation is where the observers stand back from whatever it is they are observing and do not become directly involved.

Participant observation is where the observers directly engage in the activities that they are observing such that they become a part of the interactive social context. It has been described as "a process waiting to be impressed by recurrent themes that reappear in various contexts." The type of observation which is necessary for the approach is very much determined by the social context. Natural and social contexts are more appropriate for participant observation, whilst artificial settings or a laboratory accomodate non-participant observation more easily. The emphasis throughout the remainder of this section is upon participant observation.

Deising (1971) describes participant observation as:

> "....*taking data as they come, and they usually come in scattered, disconnected fragments. Unlike the experimentalists, who can demand evidence on a specific question from his subject matter, the participant observer must adapt his thinking to what his subject happens to be doing.*

He has to observe each casual interchange as it happens, participate in the ceremony of the day since it may not occur again for two years, talk to the informants who are available, and get involved in whatever problems and controversies are prominent at the moment. At the end of the day he comes home with a wealth of information on a variety of points, but nothing conclusive on any one point. Over the weeks and months his evidence on a given point gradually accumulates and the various points start to fit together into a tentative pattern."

Advantages of Participant Observation

1. Where data or information focusing on non-verbal behaviour is required, observation studies are exceptionally useful.

2. An observer who is present in the social context where ongoing behaviour occurs can observe, interpret and make notes on the important features and events immediately.

3. Observations underlying case studies take place over an extended period of time; hence the researcher/observer has the opportunity to develop a more informal relationship with the individual

or patient and to perhaps encourage levels of empathy and rapport.

Disadvantages of Participant Observation

1. The interpretation of data or information based upon observations is generally thought to be subjective, biased, impressionistic, based upon inferences and lacking in any kind of quantitative support.

2. There is a danger of the observer becoming too much of a participant and too much involved, to the extent that he/she looses sight of his/her purposes and perspectives.

The subjective element of participant observation raises the question of external validity, for example, can the observations of a particular case or individual be extended and applied to other cases or individuals? The internal validity of participant observation, being subjective, is, on one level, more sound because it is detailed but, on another level, if the observer becomes too involved, then there is uncertainty about how representative the observations of the real individual or situation really are.

Recording Observations

One difficulty is deciding how much, and in what format, information and observational data and interpretive comments should be recorded. Note taking is one form of recording information. Wolcott (1973) comments that notes on the current observation should be fully completed before starting the next observation and procedure of note taking.

Wolcott remarks that case studies obtain certain kinds of data but do not necessarily provide the whole picture. The participant observer approach is high risk because, unless the findings can be presented in a significant and readable monograph, the only gain is experience for the researcher him/herself. The participant observer approach is also of low yield because of the considerable investment of time and personal effort. It is important, according to Wolcott, that the researcher is critical of him/herself as an instrument for collecting data through a variety of means. In effect, participant observation is best thought of as a generic term that describes a methodological approach rather than a specific method. In this sense, the case study derives essentially from a methodological approach which relies heavily upon participant observation and other selected research.

DISCUSSION POINTS

1. What type of patient might benefit from a case study, and what would the health professional gain from this approach?

2. How useful is the case study in the field of psychiatry?

USEFUL READING

Cohen, L. and Manion, L. (1980). *Research Methods in Education,* Croom Helm

Evans, K.M. (1968). *Planning Small Scale Research,* NFER Nelson

Medcof, J. and Roth, J. (1979). *Approaches to Psychology,* Open University Press

Rose, S. *et al.* (1985). *Health and Disease, U205 Course Book 1,* Open University Press

Skilbeck, M. (1983). Research methodology, *Br. Educ. Res. J.,* **9,** *1,* 11–20

Chapter 9

Triangulation

Where data or information is collected by the use of two or three research methods, it is referred to as triangulation. This multiple method attempts to explain more fully the richness and complexity of some aspect of the person, situation or event by studying it from more than one viewpoint. Triangulation is a technique for comparing and contrasting different points of view regarding a particular instance, for example the nurse's, patient's and outside observer's interpretation of the social interaction and communication taking place between nurse/patient. If it is found that the use of a questionnaire, an interview and an observational study of the same phenomena produce corresponding outcomes, then the researcher can be more confident with his/her findings (Cohen and Manion ,1980).

According to Hargreaves (1985), triangulation is an approach to research that attempts to ensure that the researchers are not imposing their own theoretical values, opinions and preferences. It is a way of checking and double checking the data and information deriving from the respondents by using several different research tools from both the quantitative and qualitative domains. It can check for consistency in what respondents say or mean, it can check that observers interpret accurately what they have observed and it can check that any numerical or statistical data is correct. These checks are provided by the use of several methods; ideally, different methods used to measure, assess or interpret the same information will yield the same kind of results.

Denzin (1970) has divided triangulation into six different types:

1. **Time triangulation** makes use of cross-sectional studies which collect data concerned with time-related processes from different groups at one particular point in time, and longitudinal studies which collect data from the same groups but at different points over a period of time. Combining these two types of studies can lessen the weaknesses and limitations that each has if used alone.

2. **Space triangulation** attemps to overcome the problem of research being culture bound. A useful criterion of research is that it is cross-cultural. For example, Levine (1966) studies achievement motivation among three Nigerian ethnic groups.

He found that the differences between the groups were not the result of the different measuring/assessment instruments, but were the result of individual and ethnic influences. He used data from a combination of dream analysis, written expressions of values and a public opinion survey for each of the three groups.

3. **Combined levels of triangulation** place emphasis upon more than one level of analysis, that is, the individual level, the interactive level (groups) and the level of collectivities (organisations, societies and cultures). Sapsford (1985) makes the comment that these levels should not be seen in any kind of hierarchical structure. Each level involves a different way of thinking about or conceptualising the same phenomena. In this sense, the different levels of analysis cannot substitute one for another; each is valid in its own right and each contributes in its own way to an understanding of a particular phenomenon. Nevertheless, Sapsford does acknowledge that levels of analysis are not absolutely distinct and, indeed, recognises that the boundaries are blurred and overlap. For example, the person requires to be understood in a social context, although the human being may

sometimes be understood out of the social context if the emphasis is simply upon his/her biochemistry.

4. **Theoretical triangulation** implies that opposing theories should be tested out through a variety of research tools. For example, rather than simply designing a questionnaire or an interview to discover how nurses perceive, value and interpret one nursing model, these research tools should be employed to find out what the nurses think about several competing theoretical models of nursing.

5. **Investigator triangulation** suggests that two or more observers/participants/researchers are involved in the study in order to compare and contrast their individual data and findings; this, inevitably, increases the validity and reliability of the research generally.

6. **Methodological triangulation** involves the use of multiple research instruments in order to indicate the degree of similarity or difference between findings.

Health care research is complex and it seems to be the case that a single-method approach yields only limited, and sometimes misleading, data and interpretation. According to Cohen and Manion (1980), for the researcher contemplating the use of triangulation, there are specific questions which need to be asked:

i) Which methods are to be selected?
ii) How are these methods to be combined?
iii) How is the information or data to be used?

These questions are very much determined by the nature of the research and the kind of information that the researcher seeks. For example, if the data are to be generalised to wider populations, then methods yielding statistical data are likely to be the most appropriate. If a researcher is particularly concerned with peoples' perceptions or conceptions (of pain or stress, for instance), then a more subjective and qualitative method, like the open-ended interview, may be more suitable. The researcher must be aware of all the possible alternative choices of methodology, their strengths and weaknesses and should ultimately select and combine those which will complement each other and build up a comprehensive picture of the nature of the research, the sample being studied and the relevance and application of the information or data generated by the subjects.

One of the biggest problems facing the researcher is that of dealing with the inconsistencies that arise from using a combination of methods, for example the differences in findings between two/three types of quantifiable methods, the differences in interpretation between two/three types of qualitative methods, and the differences when both quantitative and qualitative methods have been employed. The researcher must expect some kind of discrepancy in the data or information; a complete consensus of data is probably impossible to achieve. Nevertheless, some attempt to deal with the incongruent data must be made, for example by trying to explain or account for the differences, or by using the differences as justification for further study or additional research .

DISCUSSION POINTS

1. What combination of research methodology might you use to measure/assess:

    a) How health professionals perceive stress in their working environment?

    b) How long patients think they should remain in hospital after some particular form of surgery, and how long do health professionals think patients should be in hospital surgery?

USEFUL READING

Cohen, L. and Manion, L. (1980). *Research Methods in Education,* Croom Helm

Denzin, N.K. (1970). *The Research Act in Sociology,* Butterworth

Hargreaves, A. (1985). The micro-macro problem in sociology of education, *Issues in Education Research*, ed. Burgess, R.G. (ed.) Falmer Press

Leininger, M.M. (1985). *Qualitative Research Methods in Nursing,* Grune & Stratton

Levine, R.A. (1966). Towards a psychology of populations: the cross-cultural study of personality, *Hum. Devel.,* **3**, 30–46

Chapter 10

Critical evaluation of research articles

In health care, there are many higher-order features of the person that require better understanding in relation to care and response to illness, for example pain, compliance, stress, mental illness, communication, perception of health and illness, attitudes, quality of life, self-image, disability, grief, dying, roles, health education, cognitive ability etc. The list is obviously endless.

To carry out research in any of these areas requires that certain stages and procedures are worked through; one being a critical review of both directly and indirectly relevant previous studies carried out by other researchers. The following points are designed to facilitate a critique of research articles and papers, similar to those which appear in the *Journal of Advanced Nursing* and *Nursing Research*.

1. Has the general nature of the research problem been introduced promptly?

2. Is there a need to study the particular research problem – how far is this need supported by background knowledge and information?

3. The general problem introduced at the beginning of the article/paper should have been narrowed down to become a more specific problem – has this been done?

4. Have the concepts and terms which are to be referred to throughout the article/paper been adequately defined and explained?

5. Are the research questions/hypotheses which the researcher aims to answer clearly stated, and do they link to the specific problem that has been identified?

6. Does the article/paper sufficiently refer to previous theoretical and research literature, such that the reader feels confident that this researcher is widely read and aware of the current status of knowledge regarding both the broader and more specific areas of concern?

7. Is it made clear how this particular research will extend the knowledge generated by previous findings?

8. Is the researcher aiming to generalise the findings to a particular population – is this population clearly specified?

9. Is the sample of subjects representative of the defined population – how has the sample been selected – is the number of subjects to be involved in the study sufficient?

10. Have the notions of consent, confidentiality and rights of the subjects been dealt with?

11. Do the chosen methods of data collection match the nature of the research and the problem identified, and can they generate the kind of information that is required?

12. Has the researcher dealt with the issues of bias, reliability, validity and control over factors which may distort the research process?

13. Is the laboratory an appropriate setting for the nature of the research – OR is the social context in which the research is to be conducted representative of reality?

14. Is the data analysed appropriately and in accordance with the research methodology – were the methodological problems identified?

15. Are the findings clearly presented and discussed in terms of the research questions/hypotheses?

16. Have the findings been related to the theoretical basis of the study?

17. Has the researcher over-generalised his/her findings?

18. What are the implications for the study, and does the researcher suggest further areas for investigation?

These points, not only serve to help the health professional to critically review published research articles/papers, but they also provide guidelines for constructing and designing his/her own research. If these points are incorporated into health care research projects then less criticism is likely to be levelled at the end product.

Chapter 11

Further readings on research methods

GENERAL TEXTS

Bateson, N. (1984). *Data Construction in Social Surveys,* Allen and Unwin

Bell, C. and Roberts, H. (1984). *Social Researching: Politics, Problems, Practice,* RKP

Berger, R.M. and Patchner, M.A. (1988). *Planning for Research: A Guide for the Helping Professions,* Sage Human Services Guide

Berreman, G. (1962). *Behind Many Masks, Society for Applied Anthropology,* Monograph 4, Reprint ed A-393, Bobbs Merril

Bryman, A. (1988). Quantity and quality in social research, *Contemporary Social Research. 18,* Martin Bulmer (Series ed.) Unwin Hyman

Bryman, A. (1988). *Doing Research in Organisations,* Routledge

Bulmer, M. (1979). *Social Policy Research,* Allen and Unwin

Bulmer, M. (1986). *Sociological Research Methods,* Macmillan

Bulmer, M. (1986). *Social Science and Social Policy,* Allen and Unwin

Chapman, M. in collaboration with Basil Mahon (1986). *Plain Figures,* HMSO

de Vaus, D.A. (1986). *Surveys in Social Research,* Allen and Unwin

Eichler, M. (1988). *Non-sexist Research Methods,* Allen and Unwin

Eilon, S. (1975). Seven faces of research. *Op Res Q.* **26**, 2:ii, 359–367

Finch, J. (1986). *Research and Policy,* Falmer Press

Gardner, G. (1978). *Social Surveys for Social Planners,* The Open University Press

Grady, K.E. and Wallston, B.S. (1988). *Research in Health Care Settings,* Vol. 14, Massachusetts Institute of Behavioural Medicine

Gusfield, J. (1976). The literary rhetoric of science: comedy and pathos in drinking driver research, *Am. Soc. Rev.,* **41** (Feb), 16–34

Halfpenny, P. (1984). *Principles of Method,* Longmans

Hakim, C. (1987). research design: strategies and choices in the design of social research, *Contemporary Social Research: 13,* Martin Bulmer (Series ed.) Allen and Unwin

Hoinville, G., Jowell, R. and associates (1985). *Survey Research Practice,* Gower

Huff, D. (1954). *How to Lie with Statistics,* Pelican

Hughes, J. (1990). *The Philosophy of Social Research, 2nd edn.,* Longman

Kane, E. (1987). *Doing Your Own Research: How to do Basic Descriptive Research in the Social Sciences and Humanities,* Marion Boyars Publishers

Kurtz, N.R. (1983). *Introduction to Social Statistics,* Tokyo, McGraw-Hill

Maitland, P. and Nickals, J. (1985). *Questionnaire Design in the Probation Service: A Beginners Guide*

McRobbie, A. (1982). The politics of feminist research: between talk, text and action, *Feminist Rev.,* **12**, October

Miller, N. (1984). *A Critical Look at Value for Money, Social Science Research* From the Department of Social Administration, University of Birmingham, Vol. 3

Moore, C.M. (1987). Group techniques for idea building, *App. Soc. Res. Meth. Ser.,* Vol. 9, Sage

Morgan, D.L. (1988). Focus groups as qualitative research. *Qual. Res. Meth.,* Vol. **16,** Portland State University

Pfaffenberger, B. (1988). Microcomputer applications in qualitative research. *Qual. Res. Meth.,* Vol. **14,** University of Virginia, Charlottesville

Roberts, H. (1981). *Doing Feminist Research,* London

Rose, G. (1982). *Deciphering Sociological Research,* Macmillan

Rowbottom, R. (1977). *Social Analysis,* Heinemann

Stanley, L. and Wise, S. (??). *Breaking Out: Feminist Consciousness and Feminist Research,* RKP

Steward, D.W. (1984). *Secondary Research: Information Sources and Methods,* Vol. **4,** Sage

Thomas, P. (1985). *The Aims and Outcomes of Social Policy Research,* Croom Helm

Wenger, G.C. (1987). *The Research Relationship,* Allen and Unwin

KNOWLEDGE CREATION

Anderson, R.J., Hughes, J. and Sharrock, W.W. (1986), *Philosophy and the Human Sciences,* Croom Helm

Berger, P.L. and Luckmann, T. (1973). *The Social Construction of Reality: A Treatise in the Sociology of Knowledge,* Penguin

Cain, M. and Finch, J. (1981). Towards the rehabilitation of data, *Practice and Progress,* Abrams, P. *et al.* (eds.)Allen and Unwin

Kuhn, T.S. (1970). *The Structure of Scientific Revolutions,* University of Chicago Press

Nash, D. (1963). The Ethnologist as Stranger: An essay in the sociology of knowledge, *S.W. J. Anthropol.,* **19,** 149–167

Popper, K. (1972). *Objective Knowledge,* Clarendon Press, Oxford

Smith, D. (1973). The social construction of documentary reality. *Sociol. Enquiry*, **4**, 257–268

MAKING RESEARCH MANAGEABLE:

Formulating research hypotheses/questions

Burgess, R. (1984). *In the Field*, pp.34–38, Allen and Unwin
Burnard, P and Morrison, P. (1990). *Nursing Research in Action: Developing Basic Skills*, Macmillan
Hammersley, M. and Atkinson, P. (1983). *Ethnography: Principles in Practice*, Ch. 2, Tavistock
Kaplan, A. (1964). *The Conduct of Inquiry*, San Francisco, Chandler

Gaining access

Burgess, R. *(An Annotated Bibliography on Problems of Access)*, Ch.2 Early field experiences, *Field Research: A Sourcebook and Field Manual,*

METHODS

Evaluation research

Attkisson, C.C., Hargreaves, W.A. and Horowitz, M.J. (1978). *Evaluation of Human Service Programs,* Academic Press
Goldberg, E.M. and Connelly, N. (1981). *Evaluative Research in Social Care,* Heinemann
Hamilton, D. (1976). *Curriculum Evaluation (on service, authoritarian and democratic models of evaluation)*.Open Books

Further readings on research methods

Kosecoff, J. and Fink, A. (1982). *Evaluation Basics: A Practitioner's Manual*, Sage

Palumbo, D. J. (1988). *The Politics of Program Evaluation*, Sage

Patton, M.Q. (1988). *Utilization - Focussed Avaluation*, 2nd edn., Sage

Patton, M.Q. (1988). *Creative Evaluation*, 2nd edn., Sage

Rossi, P.H. and Williams, W. (1972). *Evaluating Social Programs: Theory, Practice and Politics*, Seminar Press

Rossi, P.H. (1985). *Evaluation and Systematic Approach*, Sage

Sandefur, G.D. (1986). *Workshop for Evaluation*, Sage

Suchman, E.A. (1967). *Evaluative Research*, Russell Sage Foundation

Wechsler, H., Reinhertz, H.Z. and Dobbin, D.D. (1976). *Social Work Research in the Human Services*, Human Sciences Press, New York

Weiss, C.H. (1972). *Evaluating Action Programs: Readings in Social Action and Education*, Allyn and Bacon, Boston, USA

Weiss, C.H. (1972). *Evaluation Research*, Prentice Hall

York, R.O. (1982). *Human Service Planning: Concepts, Tools and Methods*, University of North Carolina Press

Survey procedures/questionnaires

Babbie, E.R. (1973). *Survey Research Methods*, Wadsworth

Berdie, D.R. and Anderson, J.F. (1974). *Questionnaires: Design and Use*, Scarecrow Press

Hoinville, G. and Jowell, R. (1985). *Survey Research Practice*, Gower

Hyman, H.H. (1955). *Survey Design and Analysis*, Free Press

Marsh, C. (1983). *The Survey Method*, George Allen and Unwin

Moser, C.A. and Kalton, G. (1979). *Survey Methods in Sociological Investigation,* 2nd edn., Heinemann

Oppenheim, A.N. (1966). *Questionnaire Design and Attitude Measurement,* Heinemann

Sudman, S. and Bradburn, N.M. (1983). *Asking Questions: A Practical Guide to Questionnaire Design,* Jossey Baer

Historic Analysis

Becker, C. (1935). *Everyman His Own Historian,* New York, F.S. Crofts

Carr, E.H. (1965). *What is History?*, New York, Alfred A Knopf

Gottschalk, L. (ed.) (1945). *The Use of Personal Documents in History, Anthropology and Sociology,* New York, Social Science Research Council Bulletin 53

Lyman, Stanford (1968). Accounts. *Am. Sociol. Rev.,33, 1*

Fieldwork

General

Burgess, R. (1982). Field research: A sourcebook and field manual. *Contemporary Social Research,* Bulmer, M. (ed.) Vol.4, Allen and Unwin

Burgess, R. (1984). In the field: an introduction to field research, *Contemporary Social Research,* Bulmer, M. (ed.), Vol.8, Allen and Unwin, London

Johnson, J.M. (1975). *Doing Field Research,* The Free Press

Participant observation

Gans, H.J. (1968). the participant observer as human being: observations on the personal aspects of field work, , *Institution and the Person,* Becker, H. et al (eds.), Chicago, Aldine Publishing

Hammersley, M. and Atkinson, P. (1983). *Ethnography: Principles in Practice,* London and New York, Tavistock Publications

Schwartz, A. and Merton, D. (1973). participant observation and the discovery of meaning, *Phil. Soc. Sci.,* 1, 279–298

Sharrock, W. and Anderson, R. (1980). on the demise of the native: some observations on and a proposal for ethnography, University of Manchester, Occasional Paper No 5, December

Webster, S. (1982). Dialogue and fiction in ethnography, *Dialectical Anthropol.* 7, 2

Life history

Frank, G. (1978). finding the common denominator: a phenomenological critique of life history method. *Ethos,* 6, 4, 69–94

Langness, L.L. (1965). *The Life History in Anthropological Science,* New York, Holt Rinehart and Winston

Mandelbaum, D. (1973). The study of the life history: Ghandi, *Curr. Anthropol.* 14, 177–206

Plummer, K. (1983). Documents of life: An introduction to the problems and literature of a humanistic method, , *Contemporary Social Research*: 7, Bulmer, M. (ed.), George Allen and Unwin

Thompson, P. (1978). *Voice of the Past: Oral History,* OUP

Qualitative interviewing

Finch, J. (1984). It's great to have someone to talk to. *Social Researching*, Bell, C. and Roberts, H. (eds.),RKP

Graham, H. (1984). Surveying through stories, *Social Researching*, Bell, C. and Roberts, H. (eds.) RKP

McCrossman, L. (1984). *A Handbook for Interviewing*, HMSO (OPCS training manual)

Oakley, A. (1981). Interviewing women: A contradiction in terms. , *Doing Feminist Research*, Roberts, H. (ed.)RKP

Spradley, J. (1979). T*he Ethnographic Interview*, Holt, Rinehart and Winston

Study skills

Barzun, J. and Gratt, H. (1977). *The Modern Researcher*, (3rd edn.)

Turabian, K. (1977). *A Manual for Writers of Term Papers, Theses and Dissertations*, University of Chicago Press

Wright Mills, C. (1970). *On Intellectual Craftsmanship: An Appendix to the Sociological Imagination*, Pelican

Young, P. (1987). Writing for publication, *Nurse Educ. Today*, **7**, 285–288

Index

Action research 11, 53, 59

Case study 60, 66
Critical evaluation 74–78

Defining the research problem 23–24
Designing research 23–30

Empirical research 11
Ethical committees and codes 17, 18, 19
Ethics and research 13–22

Further readings on research methods 79–86

Generalisation 4, 5
Grounded Theory 6

Historical research 11

Interviews 25, 43–51

Non-participant observation 62

Participant observation 62–64
Patient rights 16, 18–20
Phenomenology 2, 4, 6
Philosophical research 11–12
Pilot study 26
Positivistic 3–6

Qualitative 4–9
Quantitative 2–9
Questionnaires 25, 33–42

Research methodology 24–28

Science/scientific research 2–9
Subjects in research 25

Triangulation 67–73